BECOMING OF AGE : 2
escaping the temptation and addiction of smoking

Temptations is the worst enemy of the restless teenage years. Temptations lurk around everywhere for the curious teenagers. Smoking is one of those temptations that many teenagers are hooked for life.

S.ELIA

TRIALS AND TRIBULATIONS OF GROWING UP

Self published by S .ELIA

With Kindle Direct Publishing   @ amazon.com

The uneasy restless teenage years

Temptations is the worst enemy of the restless
teenage years.
During the teenage years, many teenagers are
hooked on many dangerous to the health habits.
 Temptations lurk around every corner for the
curious teenagers.
Teenagers are anxious to grow up to prove to the
world that they arrived . In their quest to prove that

they are no longer babies or kids they fall to the temptations that the grown ups went through during their teenage years, especially smoking. Yes, it is a fact many grown ups smoke. Tobacco companies used advertisements of famous people smoking their products with the objective that ordinary people will try to mimic their idol's smoking habit . So the teenagers think that if they smoke, especially in public, people will accept them as grown ups too. That's a fallacy and a trap. Once they are hooked on smoking it will be hard to break that health destroying habit. They will not be the first and certainly not the last. Every generation of teenagers fall to the same trap of temptations and then some.

There are new fads, temptations and new addictive products introduced every year for the consumption by young and old. Some will try these new and old addictive products and will be hooked for life, and some of them will even cost them their lives. But that is the circle of life,

And that's the real temptation and thinking I had, when I was in my early teenage years...........and I was almost hooked on smoking.

My story how I dodged the smoking habit!

When I was thirteen going fourteen, I was tempted to smoke many times. As a matter of fact it was more than tempting.
I used to smoke off and on with my teenage buddies. Nothing serious but I started experimenting with smoking.
It all started when a group of friends of mine, we were playing soccer in the nearby field. It was a beautiful, sunny hot day with a breezing wind.
After the game was over we sat on the grass under a tree to rest and drink some soft drinks to cool down. One of the boys, who was a few years older than me, took a packet of cigarettes out of his pocket, took a cigarette and started smoking.

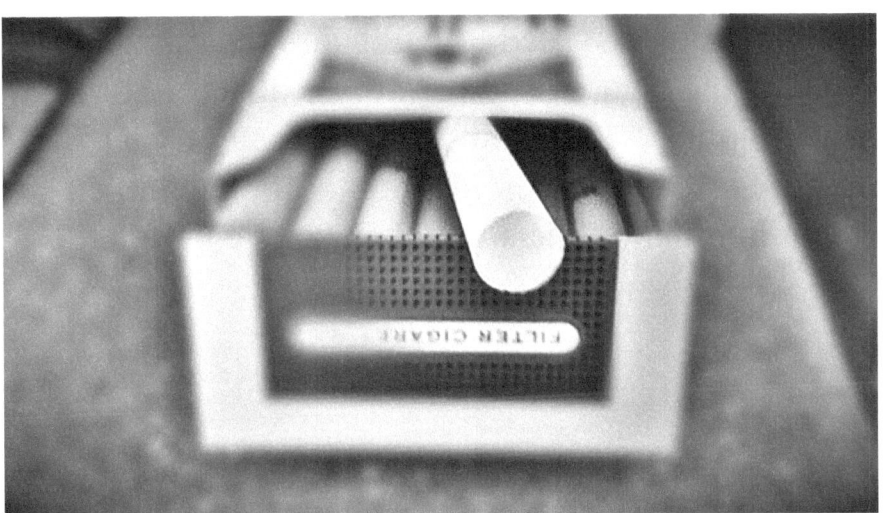
Pack of cigarettes

He offered his pack of cigarettes to the rest of the
boys. Some of them apparently were used to
smoking and they gladly accepted the cigarette and
started smoking too. Me and a few others did not
accept the offer.
 The guy with the packet of cigarettes urge the
rest of us to try smoking and he said : " common
you guys, try it , you will like it. It is fashionable to
smoke, don't you see all the famous actors
smoking and Girls like cool guys that smoke?"
I was still hesitant to try but the guy took a
cigarette out of the pack and gave it to me by
saying: "here take it, try it you'll like it."
I hesitantly took the cigarette and put it on my
mouth. The guy encourage me to take my first
smoke. He lit up my cigarette and I tried to
smoke but I choked up with severe   coughing .

The other boys started to laugh and the boy who gave me the cigarette said: "no, no, that's not the way to do it." " look and learn how to do it". He put his cigarette on his mouth, took a huge breath in inhaling the smoke from his cigarette .

He then took the cigarette out of his mouth , looked up and he let out a huge amount of smoke clouding his entire face. And he said . " you see that's the way to do it, it is so easy, try it" just put the cigarette on your mouth and take a deep breath in, inhaling   the smoke

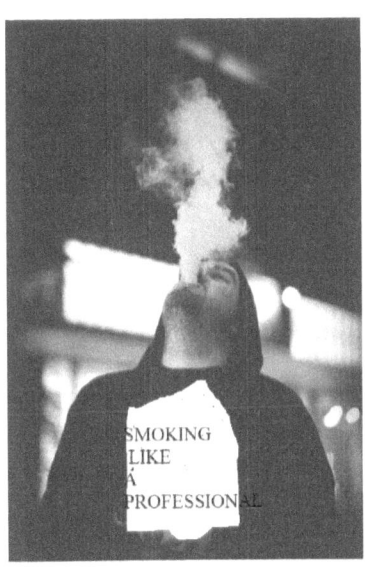

SMOKING
LIKE
A
PROFESSIONAL

from the cigarette,
and then blew the smoke out."

I did that and it was somewhat better than the first
time. The guy who gave me the cigarette said:"
there you go, with a little practice you will be good
at it, and you will like it."
I let the cigarette burn down to more than have ,
hesitantly took a last inhale in of smoke and threw
it on the ground and stepped on it to extinguish it.

Then we all headed to our homes. On the way home,, I felt that there was some smell of cigarette in my breath. Fearing that my mother will detect the smell of the cigarette smoke in my breath and get mad at me, I asked one the boys if there is anything to do to get rid of that smell.

He said:" sure , here take some mint chewing gum and the smell will disapear."

When I got home, it was time for dinner already. We had a delicious dinner, one of my mother's superb cooking .

Fortunately she did not detect any cigarette smell in my breath.

My mother was not a smoker and she disliked smoking. She was constantly telling my father who was a part time smoker, to stop burning his hard earning money smoking cigarettes.

My father used to smoke a couple of cigaretes a day and usually had a habit of smoking one cigarette   with his coffee right after dinner. . As usual, right after dinner he went out to have his coffee and smoke his cigarette.

 My mother looked at me and she whispered slowly:' I don't understand what pleasure he gets from smoking cigarettes and filling up his lungs with dirty smoke". don't you ever start smoking.'

 I   just shrugged my shoulders and said nothing. In the next few days and weeks I continued to see my buddies and kept experimenting with our new found habit, smoking. We were carefull not to smoke in public from the fear that somebody will report us to our parents. We never smoke on school premises , as the school principle had warned all the school students , that anybody caught smoking will be expelled from the school. My experimentation with smoking lasted about a year and I started to like smoking and being cool, like the rest of my buddies , as some of us thought at the time.

By the time I was fourteen years old going fifteen , I wanted to buy a bicycle. Without a bike , I used to walk or take the bus anywhere I wanted to go. I did not like that. I wanted to have my own two wheels and go everywhere I wanted to go.

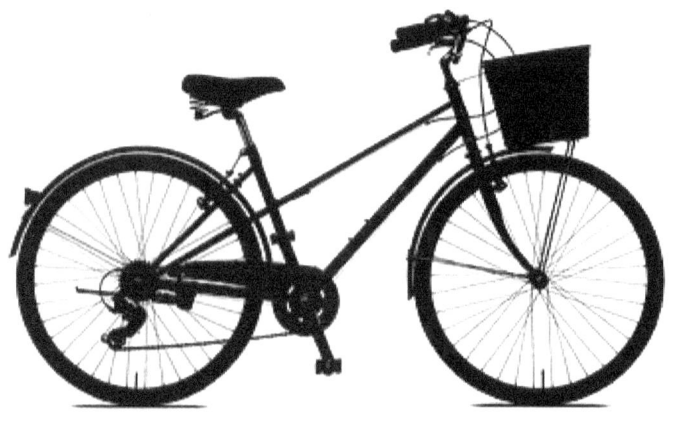

The is the bike I wanted to have, for my transportation and my freedom from walking and long waits for the bus rides.

I wanted to buy a bicycle but I did not have the money.

It was summer time , the school year was over and I had a lot of free time to do many things I liked to do . I wanted to go to the beach and swim in the waters of the calm blue sea, but without a bike it was impossible to walk to the beach, it was too far away. Taking the bus it was a long ride and the bus did not go straight to the beach.

Most of my friends had bikes and they let me use their bikes occasionally, but they used their bikes daily and it was not possible for me to borrow their bikes for any length of time.

I talked to my parents asking them to buy me a
bicycle   but they told me that they did not have
the money to buy me one at that time. But my dad
suggested that if I really wanted to buy a bicycle,
to go to work in the nearby vineyard for a few
weeks during the summer break. He said that many
kids my age work there during the summer to earn
some extra money for their needs. He finished by
saying that one of his friends was a supervisor at
the vineyard and he could   ask him to hire me
there for the summer.
I was planning to spend my summer school break,
doing all the fun things I wanted to do , like going
to the beach and playing with my friends . If I had
to work, I could not do all those fun things I liked,
but   I badly wanted to buy a bicycle so I
hesitantly said, I will try.

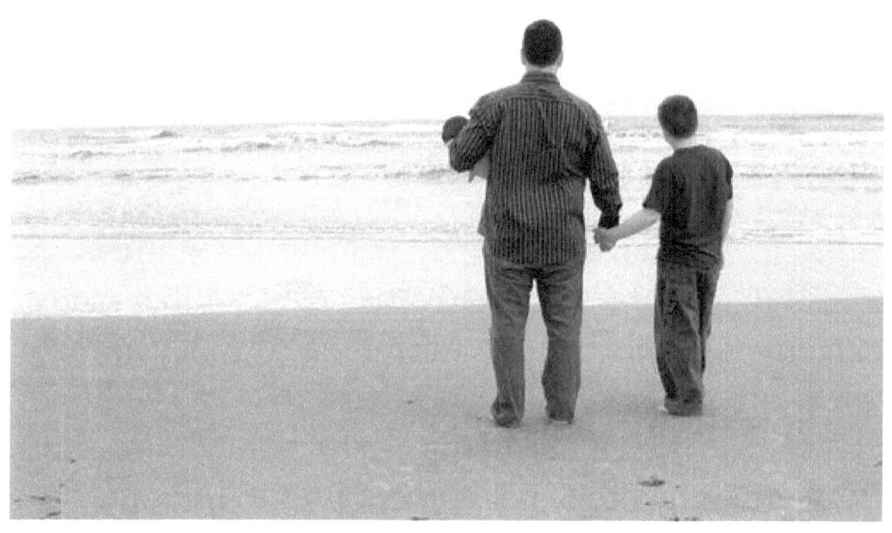

My dad called his friend and he arranged for me to start working in the vineyard. My father's friend gave him all the details how I was going to go to the vineyard and start work.

It was Saturday afternoon and I was supposed to be in the vineyard on Monday morning by seven o'clock, by taking the vineyards bus and meeting the supervisor at vineyards office.

Working in the vineyard.

The vineyard was a huge place with thousands of acres of different types of grape plants, orange groves, tangerines, grapefruits and avocado. They also had a big storage and packaging facility for their fruits.

They had their regular workers working to cultivate, fertilize, prune and keep the plants in good healthy condition.

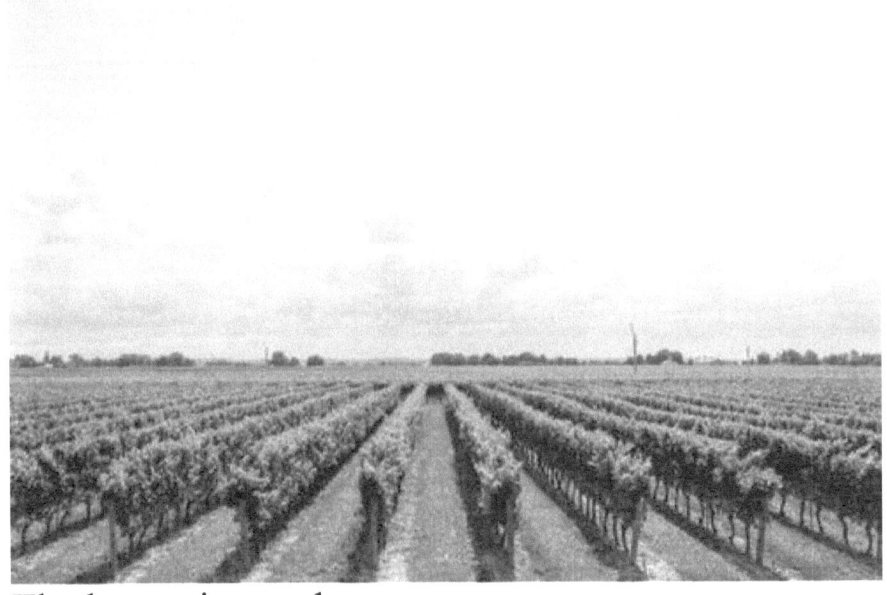

The huge vineyard .

During the harvest period the company hired temporary workers, including many youngsters during their summer school break to help out the regular workers .

It was summer time and it was time to harvest the first ripe sultana grapes and my father arranged with his friend who worked for many years in the vineyard , to hire me to help out the regular workers.

On Monday, as it was arranged by my father and his supervisor friend, I went to the vineyard with one my friends and we started working in the storage and packaging facility of the company helping the women that worked there packaging the ripe sultana grapes for export and the local market. The job was quite easy and as a matter of fact I enjoyed working there for five weeks. Everyday we had lunch time from eleven to eleven thirty and we finished the day's work at five o'clock in the afternoon . Just outside the packing facility there were some picnic tables and we were sitting there during the lunch time with my new found teenage friends that worked there for the summer.

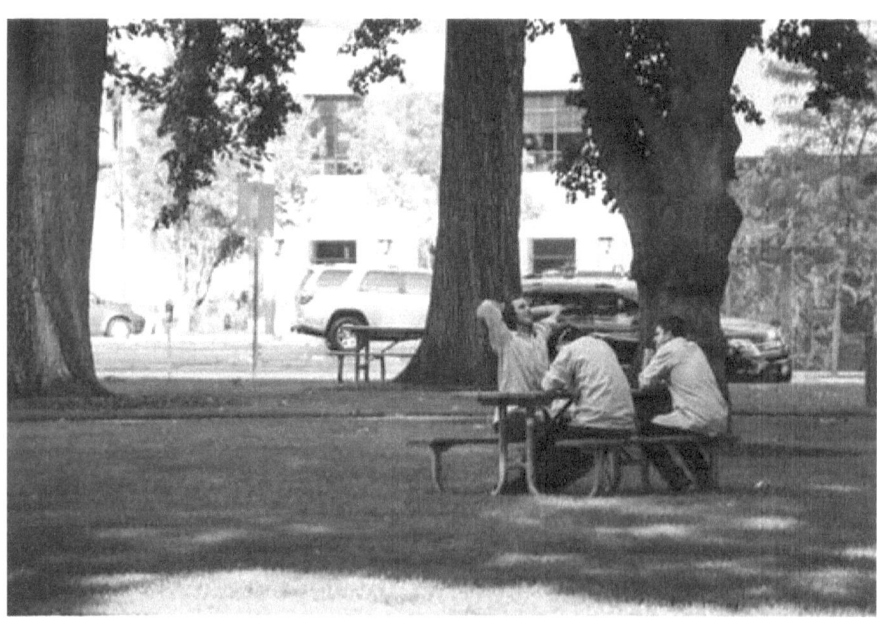

Beside us there were other tables and other workers were having their lunch.

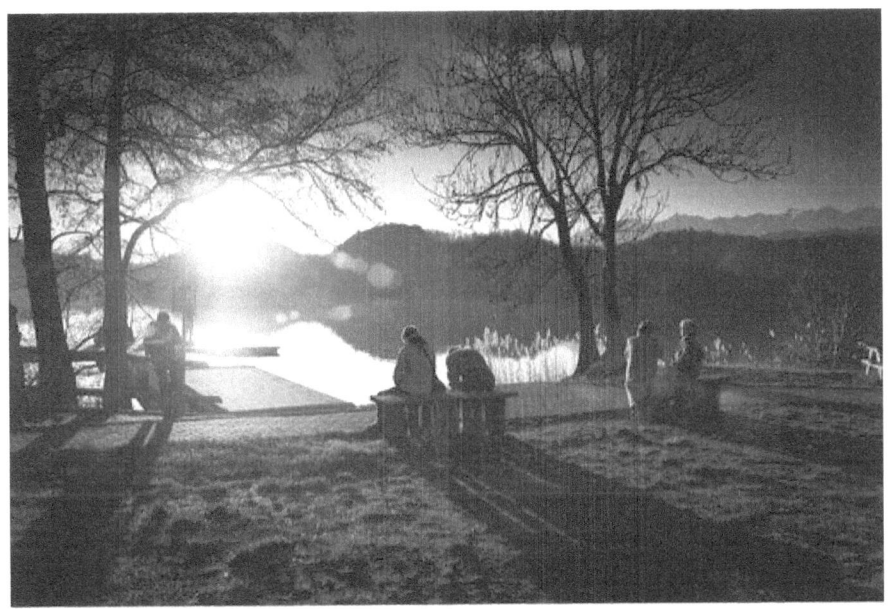

During one of those lunch breaks, there were two regular older workers having their lunch in the next picnic table from our picnic table.
One of the regular workers told the other one that he went to see their co-worker who was sick in the hospital with cancer. He went on to describe his sick co-workers condition, that he was in a terrible pain, hooked up in some respirator machines and having difficulty in breathing and coughing constantly. He finished by saying that his prognosis was not good and the doctors told his family that even with surgery his chances for survival were

not good.

The other worker , nodded and he said, "I know, I know that very well. My poor father had the same condition and he suffered so much pain and discomfort in the last three months of his life. The pain medications did not help him much, he was in constant pain, coughing and he had difficulty in breathing. He was staying with us at the time and my wife and kids were worrying about his condition.

His death was a relief to his suffering and a warning to all those who smoke that they can have the same suffering. That's why I gave up smoking. I used to smoke a pack of cigarettes a day but my wife and kids urged me to give up smoking . I remember vividly my younger daughter, she was seven at that time, looking in my eyes with her beautiful brown eyes and saying: please dad stop smoking. I do not want you to die like grandpa. I love you dad and I want you to be here with our family. Please daddy stop smoking".

After that emotional plea from my young daughter, and thinking about my wife and all my kids, I threw the packet of cigarettes in the fireplace that was burning at the time and I quit smoking . It has been ten years since my dad had such a painful end and I never smoked another cigarette again.

My three kids after seeing their grandpa suffering

so much, they never even want to hear the word "smoke". None of them smoke and they cannot even stand if someone else smoke in their presence. They usually tell them the tragic end of their grandpa who used to smoke two packs of cigarettes a day and he was considered to be the leader of smokers of his time.
The other co-worker said: "good for them, they are smart kids, you should be proud of them."
The co-worker with the non smoking kids said:" yes , I am very proud of my kids , and I am very thankful that they made me quit smoking too. I feel so much better without the smoking.!"

The lunch break was over and we all returned to work, but I could not forget what I just heard the two workers talking about their co worker and the painful end of the other coworker's father.

Listening to that made me thinking that smoking was not cool and glamorous after all, but just a bad habit that could lead to serious diseases, like cancer. Although I was used to smoking one or two cigarettes a day like my dad, I decided to stop smoking altogether from fear that something bad can happen to my health from the smoking. I still had a few cigarettes in my hiding place, I took them out, crumbled them up and threw them in the garbage.

Next time we had a gathering with the other teenage friends of my neighborhood and they started to smoke I told them about the story I heard from the old coworkers in the vineyard, and my decision not to smoke again. Some of them laughed and some of them were skeptical but I told them that I made my decision and I was not going to smoke again.

 The guy that gave me the first cigarette and the first lesson in smoking , he laughed and said :" we will see, before long you will want to be cool again and you will start smoking."

I said: "getting sick is not cool, besides I will be saving my money for other useful things , like buying my first bicycle, and that is better than burning my money   smoking cigarettes."

He said: " good for you man, but will see."

After working for five weeks in the vineyard , the sultana harvest was over and I had enough money to buy my first bicycle.

 I went with my dad   to a bicycle store and I bought the bike I wanted. That bike gave me the freedom from walking , taking the bus to school, going to movies and everywhere else I wanted to

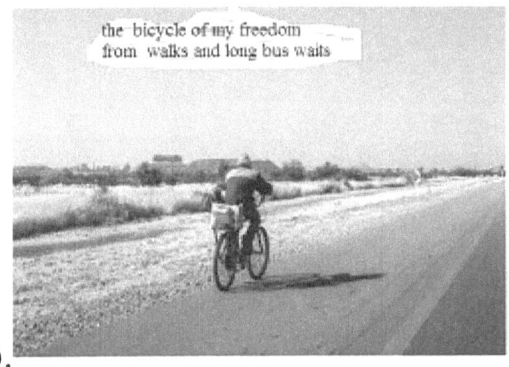

the bicycle of my freedom
from walks and long bus waits

go.

Just before going back to school after the summer
break, me and my friend who also had a bicycle ,
we went to the movies to see one of   007 agent ,
Sean's Connery movies .
In the movie theatre were some other boys I knew
including that guy who gave me my first
cigarette. During the movie most of the people
were smoking including some of the boys I knew.
Before long the movie theatre was full of thick
smoke from all the smoking .

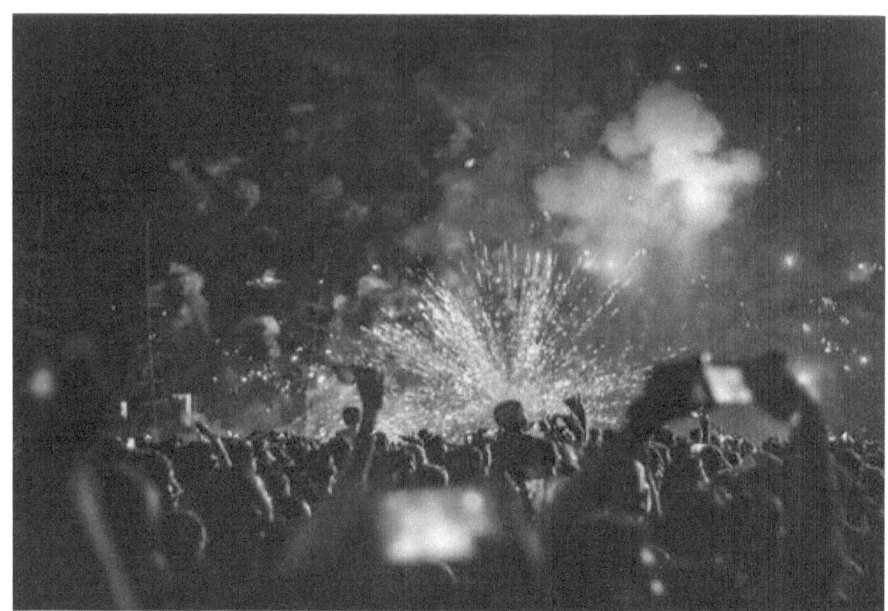

Smoked filled movie theatre

My clothes and hair were smelling cigarette smoke. When we got out of the movie theatre , that guy who gave me my first cigarette approached me and smiling he said:" I thought you said you were going to quit smoking." he smelled my clothes and he said: "even your clothes are smoking now." inside that movie theatre you inhaled   more smoke than ten packs of cigarettes!"
 I looked at him and shrugged my shoulders and I said: " you are probably right , that's why I will give up going to places that are full of cigarette smoke."
While pedaling back home with my brand new bicycle I started to cough and had a mild pain in

my chest. I was scared that my lungs were damaged from all that smoke I breathed inside that movie theatre.

When I reached home I told my mom about my pain ,my cough and my fears that something might be wrong with my lungs.

She said : " son, I will take you to the emergency department to see what the doctor has to say".

We went to the nearest emergency department and after a short time waiting the nurse took me to have some chest x-rays and then she took me and my mother to see the doctor on duty.

The doctor was a middle aged man with thick glasses and a friendly face.

He looked at my x-rays, then he examined my throat for my cough and listened to my chest with his stethoscope. He then asked me in front of my mother if I was smoking. I said:" no but I was in the movie theatre and It was full of other people smoking and unfortunately I had to breath in all that smoke."

He said: " I see, that explains why you smell tobacco and your clothes have the smoking smell. Your lungs are clear but you have a cold and with all that smoke made things worse.'

I asked the doctor if my lungs were damaged from all that smoke I had to breath in the movie theatre.

After that, the doctor called the nurse and ask her to brink some x-rays. The doctor put the x-rays on a view box and he turned to me and my mother and he said." the first x-rays are your x-rays and look good, no damage is present in your lungs. The second x-rays are from a patient that smoked cigarettes all his life and he was having all sorts of lung problems. You see what smoking can do to the lungs of people who smoke? He pointed out the dark area of the x-rays of the lungs and he said: " this man died from lung cancer last week. That's how smoking destroys the lungs of people. "

"Perhaps this unpleasant scare you had with your chest pain to day , will teach you a lesson about the dangers of smoking. I hope that you are a smart boy and you will not take up the deadly habit of smoking."

. Take this cough medicine and you will be fine in a couple of days, and Avoid any area with smoking." smoking can cause serious damage to the lungs".

My mother thanked the kind doctor about his services and good advice and we left the hospital . My mother and I were relieved that I had a cold and it was not anything else more serious. She turned to me and she said :" you heard the doctor what he said about smoking, don't you ever try smoking, I wished your father stopped smoking too."

In a few days I was feeling very good and it was time to return to school for another school year. I never went to the movies again and I preferred to watched television at home. I kept seeing my buddies and some of them still were smoking but I had nothing to do with smoking any more.

Working in that vineyard during the summer school break to save money for my first bicycle, taught me valuable lessons about working, saving money and the importance to eliminate my bad smoking habit.

That working experience I had when I was fourteen going fifteen had a tremendous influence on my life.

Thinking back, I am glad that my parents did not just buy me the bicycle I wanted, but instead they let me earn the money I needed for that bicycle. It taught me valuable lessons that no amount of money can ever teach me.

Ever since that story I heard about the deadly consequences of smoking and my scare with chest pain, and the trip to that emergency room , I never smoked again, and I cannot even stand the smoke when others smoke. In short that working experience saved me from the deadly habit of smoking.

__Never mind the money I saved form not smoking but it also saved my life from a dangerous habit of smoking and you cannot put a price on that.__

Over the years the attitude towards smoking has changed dramatically. People changed the way they see smoking. No longer people think that smoking is cool or glamorous, mainly due to education about the harmful effects of smoking. They also made new laws to protect the non-smokers so that no longer people can smoke in public places, restaurants

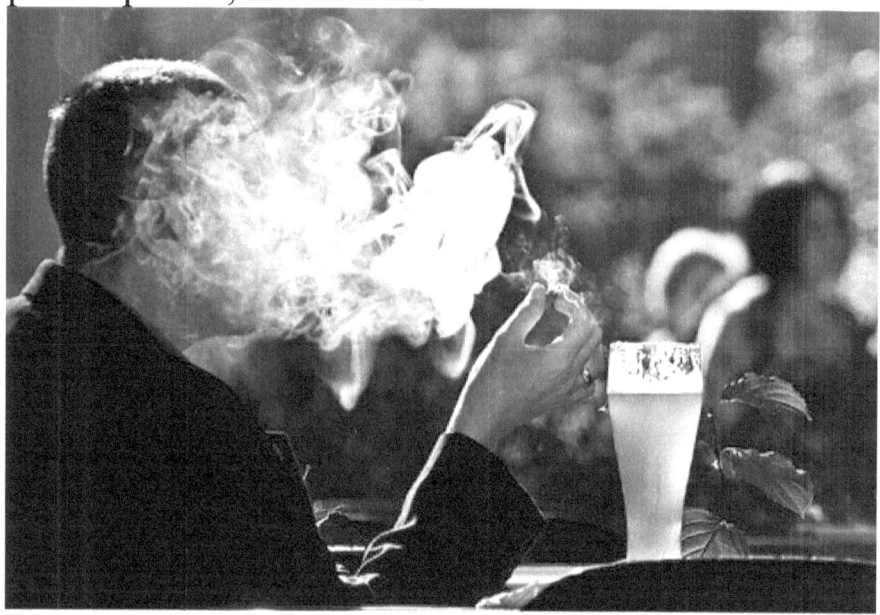

No smoking is allowed in restaurants and bars

like movies, grocery stories, government buildings , the planes, buses,

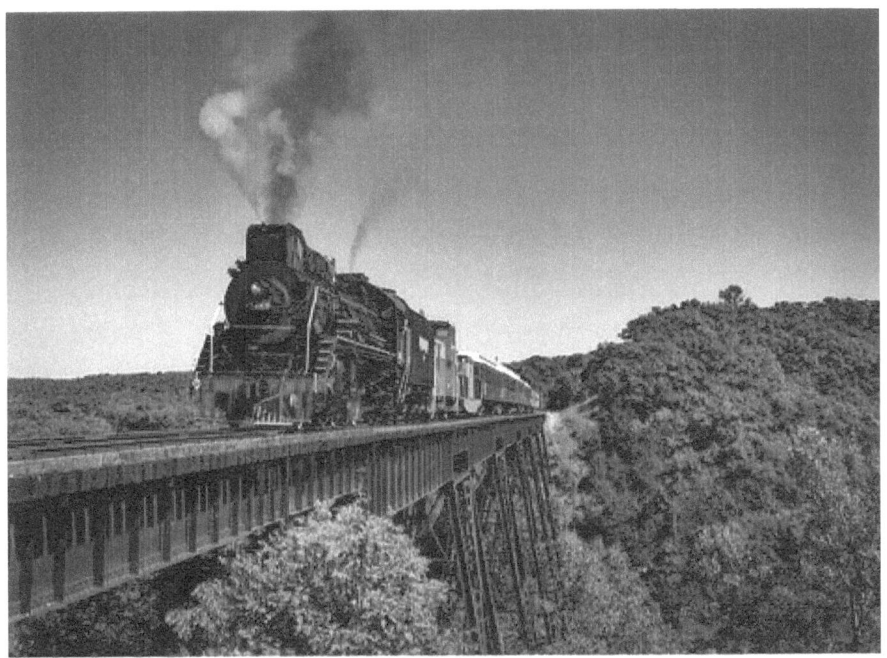

No smoking in trains or   buses

trains or even coffee shops. That is progress   in a good way to protect peoples lives from the deadly effects of smoking.

Lets see what are the benefits if any, and the harmful   effects of smoking.

Ths harmful effects of smoking.

Smoking is a dangerous habit that causes damage to the lungs.

The lungs job is to receive fresh oxygenated fresh air and take the oxygen for the body's needs and remove carbon monoxide from the body . The Oxygen provides the body with energy, while carbon dioxide is a bodily waste produced by cellular metabolism that collects in the tissues of the body and is removed by the lungs.

When the fresh air enters the lungs does not cause any damage to the lungs. However when smoke from cigarette or any other type of smoke enter the lungs it causes damage to the lining of the lungs and eventually it makes them dark and diseased and unable to do the proper oxygen/ carbon dioxide exchange. It is like the chimney , the more smoke go through the chimney the darker and charred becomes and eventually blocks the chimney.

So the damage to lungs depends how much smoked is inhaled by the smoker.

The list of diseases caused by smoking are: emphysema, Chronic Bronchitis, Asthma, Cardiovascular Diseases Cancer, Stroke. Peptic Ulcers, Atherosclerosis Diabetes, skin problems, smokers wrinkles, fertility problems, premature aging and many other conditions.

The health professionals that treat smokers, know

that smoking only damage can cause to the lungs, and no health benefit at all.

Smoking causes lung damage, including cancer, damage to the heart and heart vessels . Smoking can also cause damage to the reproductive system and problems with reproduction to both males and females.

Smoking is an addiction and people that are addicted to the nicotine of the cigarettes have difficulty to quit.

Are there any health benefits from smoking any type of smoke ?

The short answer is no.

However do not be surprised if you find people, even some in the so called scientific community that will say that there are benefits in smoking. One such claim is that smoking helps, loose weight, stress relief, and that smoking lowers the risk of knee-replacement surgery. Just wondering what type of smoke they were smoking when they make such claims?

There was even a lawyer for the tobacco companies that he suggested   that smoking is good because people die early and save the governments from paying them pensions,   drug and medical benefits.

Just wondering what he was smoking when he made such statements on national television? No matter what some people will try to say that there are benefits when smoking, it is just their personal theory without any supporting facts. The millions of people that suffer from the detrimental dangerous effects of smoking, prove that smoking is a very dangerous habit causing many diseases. Ultimately people can make their own choices and decisions about their lives, and if they decide to smoke, they are free to make that choice.

Vaping

Many people addicted to long term smoking are trying to quit smoking by switching to vaping. Vaping is a new mechanical device invented in the last two decades and was considered as safer alternative to smoking.

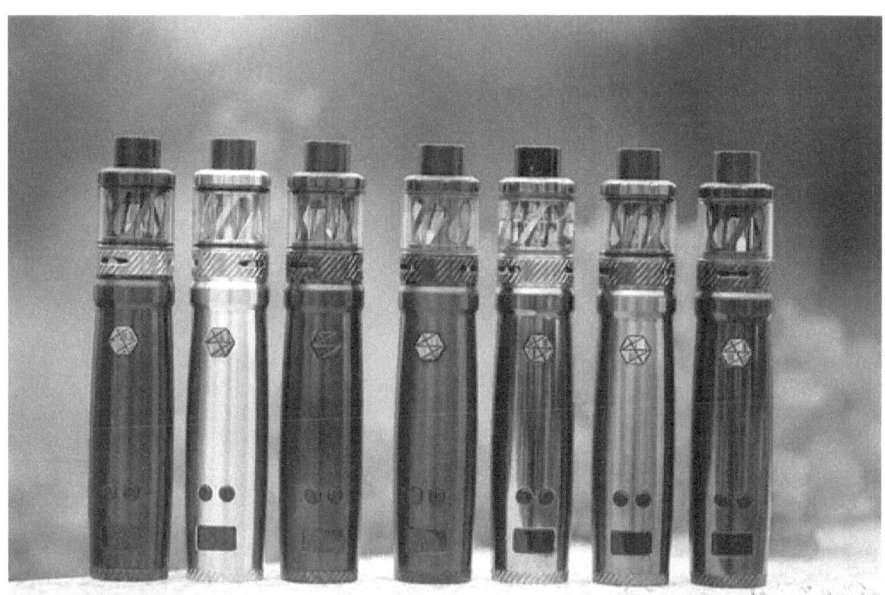

Vaping devices

Vaping is the act of inhaling and exhaling an aerosol produced by a vaping product, such as an electronic cigarette. Vaping doesn't require burning like cigarette smoking. The device heats a liquid into a vapor, which then turns into aerosol. This vapor is often flavored and can contain nicotine.

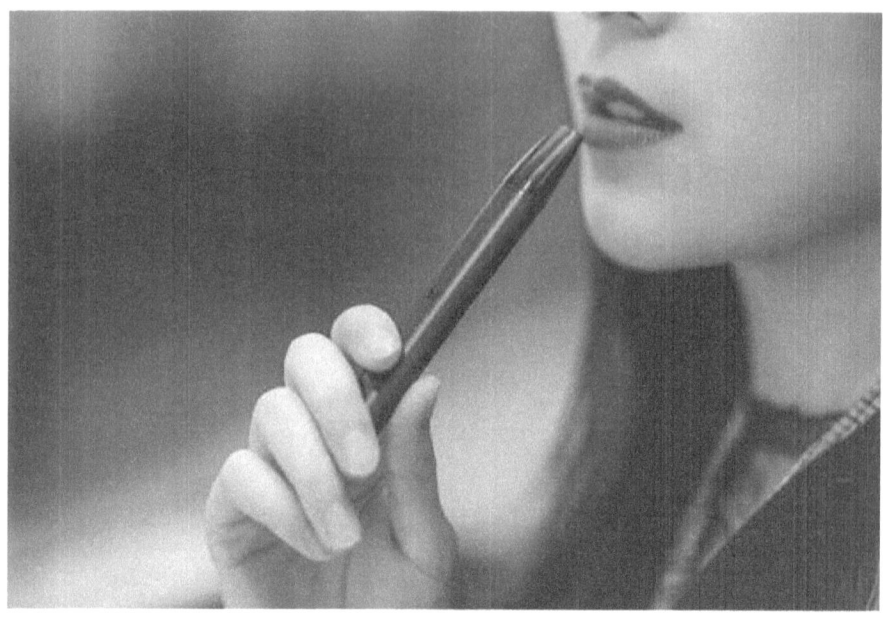

Vaping devices are usually battery-powered. They may come with removable parts. Vaping products have many names, and are produced by different manufacturers.

Many people managed to quit smoking but now they are addicted to vaping thus replacing one addiction with another not necessarily a healthier choice.

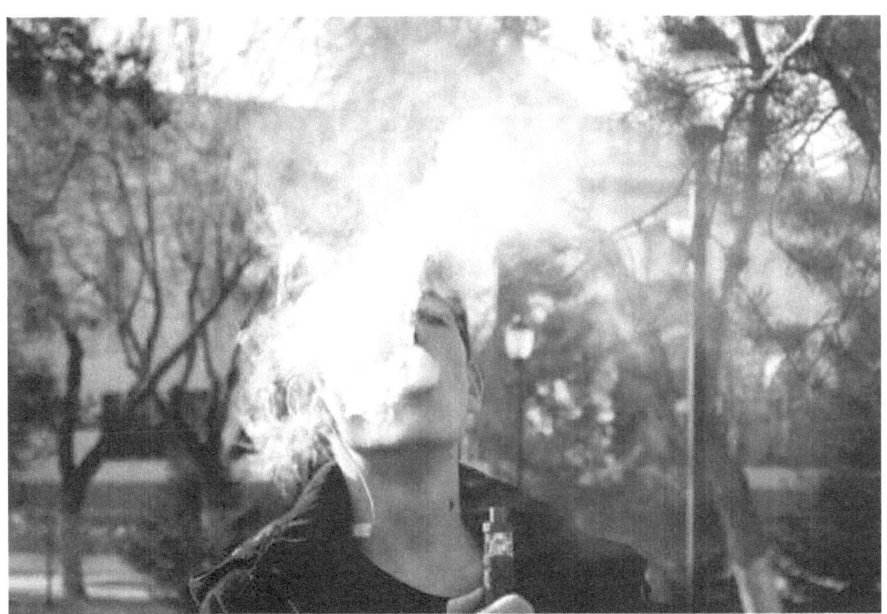

A man using his vaping device

Although people thought that vaping was less harmful than cigarettes smoking, the latest news indicated that many people suffered severe lung damage from vapimg and some of them died. That forced the governments to put strict restrictions   on the sales of vaping and make new regulations about vaping .

Other types of smoking.

There are many other types of smoking besides

cigarettes smoke, depending on the preferences of the smoker.

Many people smoke marihuana claiming that it is better than smoking cigarettes and that it has medicinal properties .

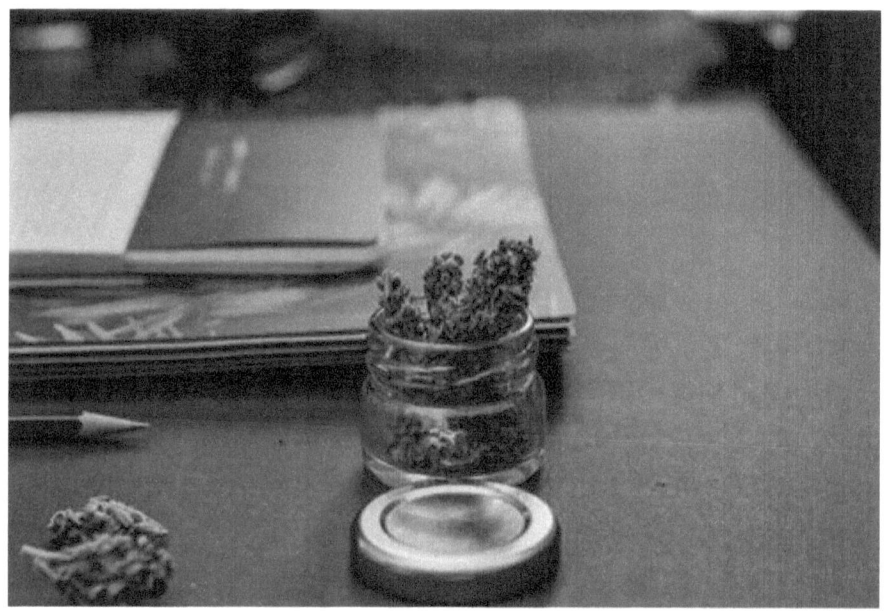

Marihuana used by many for smoking

Some other people they prefer to smoke cigars which is also made from the tobacco plant like the cigarettes

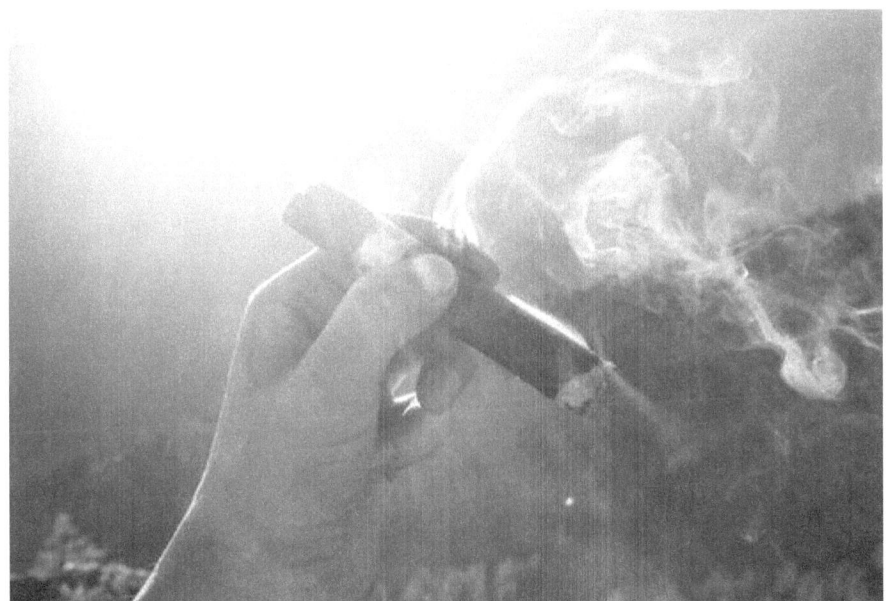

The cigar produced mainly in Cuba is popular by many smokers, but it does not mean that it is better that any other type of smoke, or less risky for your health.

Other people smoke pipes

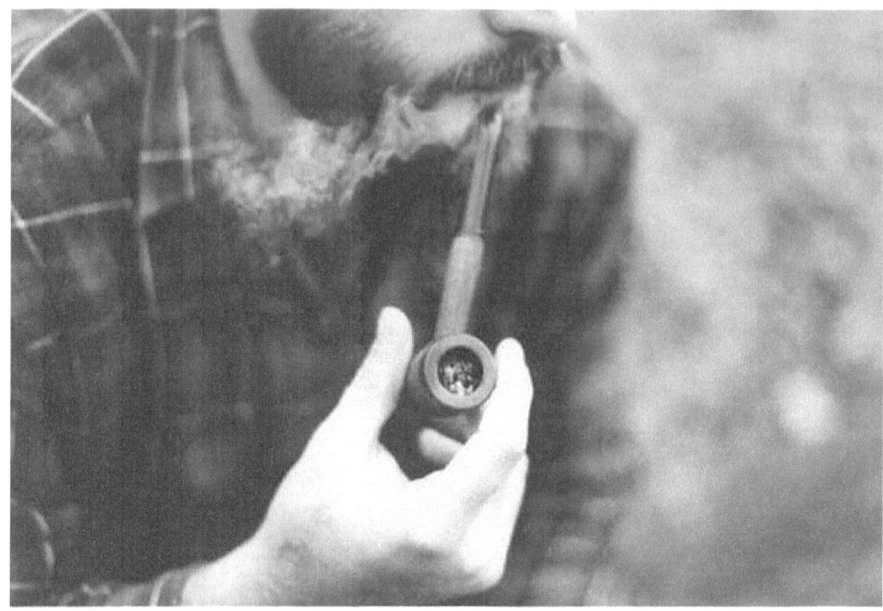

People smoking pipes claim that is less dangerous to their health that cigarettes smoking , but that depends entirely how much and how often they smoke.

Other people prefer to smoke hookahs, but this type of smoking can be more dangerous than other types of smoking as the charcoal that heats the tobacco produces large quantities of harmful carbon monoxide and heavy metals as well as nicotine, thus causing more harm to the lungs.

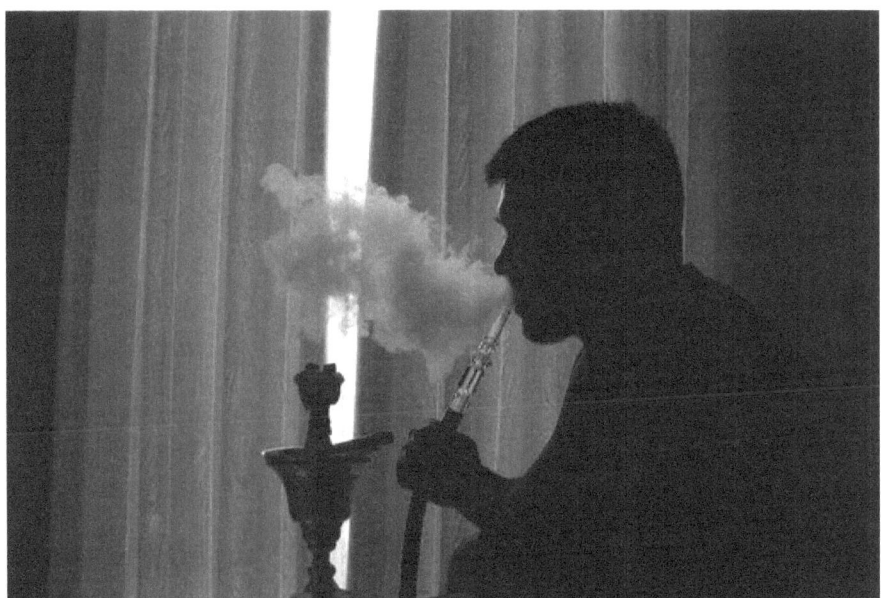

Tobacco in hookahs is heated by charcoal.

Other people prefer to smoke herbs and other substances. But no matter what they smoke is still harmful to their health.

__The lungs were made to breath in fresh air for the body's oxygen needs and expel out the body's waste carbon dioxide and mot to inhale polluted smoke from any source! In Many house fires, people die from smoke inhalation and not the fire itself!__

Conclusion

When I was thirteen going fourteen I did not know much about the health risks of smoking . Being a teenager and easily persuaded that smoking is a cool thing to do , I tried smoking for a short period of time.

 In a way, I was fortunate to hear   the sad stories of other people suffering from the harmful effects of smoking.

 The scare I had after breathing second hand smoke in a movie theatre , made me decide not only to never smoke again, but also avoid   second hand smoke anywhere there were people smoking.

When I was young, I did not know much about the different types of smoking and the harmful effects on the lungs, but now that I do know, I think I made the best decision for me.

Any type of smoke from tobacco products, marihuana, herbs or any other type smoke including the fireplace smoke, causes damage to the lungs. Smoke is produced by a chemical reaction when you burn something, creating a chemical reaction called combustion. The combustion process produces toxic gasses that are harmful to your lungs and the whole body. Those toxic gasses destroy the lungs and they loose the ability to supply the body with fresh oxygen needed and expel the carbon dioxide that the body does not need.

All people smoking tobacco products have huge health risks and none is safer than the other. All contain harmful substances that create toxic chemicals when they burn and most also contain a highly addictive drug, nicotine.

The only way to reduce and completely eliminate the risk to your health is by quitting smoking altogether and not substituting one bad habit with another equally harmful smoking habit.
__All smoking habits cause charring harm to the lungs making them look like a used chimney.__
The best way to avoid the health risks from smoking is to never start smoking and avoid any places that other people smoke and even avoid any smoke from any source including your barbecue or fireplace.

If you are a smoker, the best thing you can do for your health and the health of your kids, family and others is to quit smoking altogether.

In conclusion, there are no benefits from smoking any type of smoke, only damaging your health and your pocket with your hard earned money going up in smoke! You can replace your money but unfortunately you cannot repair your health!

IF IT IS POSSIBLE, STOP SMOKING TO-DAY, NOT TOMORROW, NOT NEXT WEEK.
The best time to quit smoking is now.
DO IT FOR YOUR HEALTH
 DO IT FOR THE HEALTH OF YOUR KIDS AND FAMILY
DO IT FOR THE ENVIROMENT AND THE HEALTH OF OTHERS.
Ultimately the final decision is up to you to make your own choices and decisions...........

References.

All the pictures are from the internet from the websites of pexels and
Pixabay which clearly state: .pictures from their websites may be used freely for almost any purpose - even commercially.
 Attribution is appreciated, but not required.

From the inside cover.

After reading this book and you no longer need it, give it to someone else to benefit from the writings in this book.
Knowledge is to be shared for the benefit all, and that is the main reason for witting books: to convey information.
 If you find the knowledge in this book helpful , write a good review of this book,
 or recommend it to others to learn that work is good for your pocket .

The author

The author is a retired health professional interested in health issues, fitness, exercises, nutrition and other lifestyle topics.
In this book he writes about his own personal story, how he managed to avoid the addiction of smoking after he accidentally heard the tragic stories of other people affected by the addiction of smoking.
It is the personal belief of the author that smoking any type of smoke is bad for your health and your pocket.

For the back cover

This book is about the personal experiences of the

author about the troubles and tribulations of the teenage years , when he was growing up.

This book is bout the personal philosophy of the author about smoking..

Read this book to learn the health risks of smoking.

Read this book to learn the many health risks of smoking.

Or just read this book out of curiosity to see how the author managed to dodged the smoking habit.

Buy this book as a gift to your teenage kids to learn that smoking is never cool and it is bad for their health.

www.ingramcontent.com/pod-product-compliance
Lightning Source LLC
Chambersburg PA
CBHW030539220526
45463CB00007B/2896